The MINDFUL Path to Success

Michel Montalvo

Table of Contents

Part I: The Foundation
Chapter 1
Introduction to Mindfulness and Success

Mindfulness, often associated with ancient Eastern philosophies, has gained significant traction in recent years as a powerful tool for enhancing personal and professional success. At its core, mindfulness is the practice of being fully present in the moment, observing thoughts and feelings without judgment.
By cultivating this awareness, individuals can unlock their full potential and experience greater fulfillment in all aspects of life.

Historically, mindfulness practices have been integrated into various spiritual and philosophical traditions, such as Buddhism and Hinduism.

These practices have been used for centuries to promote inner peace, reduce stress, and enhance overall well-being. In recent decades, mindfulness has emerged as a secular practice, attracting the attention of psychologists, neuroscientists, and business leaders alike.

The connection between mindfulness and success is rooted in its ability to improve cognitive functions, emotional intelligence, and overall mental health. Individuals can increase their attention span, reduce stress, and boost creativity by training the mind to focus on the present moment.

These benefits translate into enhanced performance in the workplace, improved relationships, and greater personal satisfaction.

Chapter 2
The Science
of Mindfulness

Mindfulness once considered a mystical practice, is now backed by a growing body of scientific research. Neuroscientists and psychologists have delved into the workings of the mind to uncover the mechanisms behind mindfulness's transformative effects.

The Brain's Plasticity and Mindfulness

One of the most fascinating aspects of the human brain is its remarkable ability to change and adapt, a phenomenon known as neuroplasticity. When we practice mindfulness, we're essentially training our brains to form new neural connections.

Regular mindfulness meditation has been shown to increase the thickness of the prefrontal cortex, the area of the brain responsible for decision-making, problem-solving, and emotional regulation.

Neural Pathways
and Mindfulness

Mindfulness also influences the brain's neural networks. By focusing attention on the present moment, we activate specific neural pathways that promote calmness, clarity, and focus.

This can lead to a reduction in stress hormones like cortisol, which can negatively impact our physical and mental health.

The Default Mode Network and Mindfulness

The default mode network (DMN) is a network of brain regions that are active when our minds are wandering or daydreaming. While the DMN is essential for self-reflection and future planning, excessive activity in this network can contribute to anxiety, depression, and rumination. Mindfulness meditation has been shown to reduce activity in the DMN, allowing us to be more present and less caught up in negative thoughts.

By understanding the science behind mindfulness, we can appreciate its profound impact on our well-being. It's not just a fleeting trend; it's a powerful tool that can help us live more fulfilling and meaningful lives.

Chapter 3
Mindful Focus

In today's fast-paced world, distractions are ubiquitous. From the constant ping of notifications to the allure of social media, it can be challenging to maintain focus and productivity. Mindfulness offers a powerful antidote to this pervasive problem.

The Power of Focused Attention

Mindfulness is all about training our minds to focus on the present moment. By cultivating focused attention, we can improve our ability to concentrate, learn, and problem-solve.
When we're fully present, our minds are less likely to wander, and we can complete tasks more efficiently.

Techniques for Mindful Focus

Several techniques can help us enhance our focus and concentration:

- Mindful Breathing: By paying attention to the sensation of breath, we can anchor our minds to the present moment.
- Meditation: Regular meditation practice can strengthen our ability to focus and reduce mind wandering.
- Time Management Techniques: Using techniques like the Pomodoro Technique can help us break down tasks into manageable chunks and maintain focus.

Mindful Work Habits: Creating a clutter-free workspace, setting clear goals, and taking regular breaks can improve focus.

The Science of Focused Attention

Research has shown that mindfulness can increase attention span and reduce mind wandering. By practicing mindfulness, we can strengthen the neural connections associated with attention and focus. This can lead to improved performance in various areas of life, from academics to work to relationships.

By incorporating mindfulness into our daily lives, we can unlock our full potential and experience the benefits of a focused and productive mind.

Chapter 4
Creativity Unleashed

Creativity, the spark that ignites innovation and problem-solving, often seems elusive. However, mindfulness can be a powerful tool for unlocking our creative potential. By calming the mind and opening our awareness, we can tap into a wellspring of inspiration.

The Mindful Approach to Creativity

Mindfulness encourages us to approach creative tasks with a fresh perspective. When we're present in the moment, we're less likely to be constrained by rigid thinking patterns or self-doubt. Instead, we can allow our minds to wander freely, exploring new ideas and possibilities.

Practical Techniques
for Creative Mindfulness

1. Mindful Observation: Pay attention to the details of your surroundings. Observe shapes, colors, and textures. This can inspire new ideas and perspectives.
2. Mindful Breathing: Deep, intentional breathing can calm the mind and promote creativity.
3. Mindful Walking: A simple walk in nature can stimulate creativity. Pay attention to the sights, sounds, and smells around you.
4. Mindful Journaling: Write freely without judgment. This can help you explore your thoughts and feelings and uncover hidden insights.
5. Mindful Art: Engage in creative activities like painting, drawing, or music. Let your imagination flow without self-criticism.

The Science Behind Creative Mindfulness

Research suggests that mindfulness can enhance creativity by increasing divergent thinking, a cognitive process that involves generating multiple ideas. When we're in a state of mindfulness, our minds are more flexible and open to new possibilities.

By incorporating mindfulness into our creative process, we can unlock our full potential and bring our most innovative ideas to life.

Chapter 5
Emotional Intelligence and Mindfulness

Emotional intelligence, the ability to understand and manage our own emotions as well as the emotions of others, is a crucial skill for success in both personal and professional life. Mindfulness can significantly enhance our emotional intelligence by helping us develop self-awareness, self-regulation, empathy, and effective communication.

The Link Between Mindfulness and Emotional Intelligence

- Self-Awareness: Mindfulness allows us to tune into our emotions as they arise, without judgment. By observing our thoughts and feelings, we can gain a deeper understanding of ourselves.

- Self-Regulation: Mindfulness techniques, such as meditation and deep breathing, can help us manage our emotions effectively. We can learn to respond to challenges with calm and composure, rather than reacting impulsively.

- Empathy: By practicing mindfulness, we can develop a greater capacity for empathy. We can better understand the perspectives and feelings of others, leading to stronger relationships.

- Effective Communication: Mindfulness can improve our communication skills by helping us listen actively and respond thoughtfully. We can express ourselves clearly and assertively, while also being sensitive to the needs of others.

Practical Tips for Enhancing Emotional Intelligence

- Mindful Self-Reflection: Take time each day to reflect on your emotions and thoughts.
- Practice Active Listening: Pay full attention to the speaker, without interrupting.
- Develop Empathy: Put yourself in the shoes of others and try to understand their perspective.
- Practice Self-Compassion: Treat yourself with kindness and understanding.
- Mindful Communication: Express yourself clearly and assertively, while also being mindful of your tone and body language.

By incorporating mindfulness into our daily lives, we can cultivate emotional intelligence and build stronger, more fulfilling relationships.

Chapter 6: Enhancing Decision-Making

Decision-making is a fundamental human activity that impacts every aspect of our lives. However, often our decisions are clouded by biases, emotions, and impulsive thinking. Mindfulness offers a powerful tool for improving our decision-making skills.

Mindfulness and Decision-Making

Mindfulness helps us approach decision-making with a clear and focused mind. By being present in the moment, we can avoid rushing into decisions or relying on automatic responses. Instead, we can take the time to weigh our options carefully and consider the potential consequences.

Key Strategies for Mindful Decision-Making

1. Pause and Reflect: Before making a decision, take a moment to pause and reflect on the situation.
2. Gather Information: Collect all relevant information and consider multiple perspectives.
3. Consider Your Values: Align your decisions with your core values and long-term goals.
4. Trust Your Intuition: While it's important to gather information, don't underestimate the power of intuition.
5. Accept Uncertainty: Embrace the fact that not all decisions will have perfect outcomes.

By practicing mindfulness, we can make more informed and rational decisions that align with our values and goals.

Chapter 7 Reducing Stress and Avoiding Burnout

In today's fast-paced world, stress and burnout have become increasingly common. Mindfulness offers a powerful antidote to these challenges. By cultivating a sense of calm and focus, we can reduce stress, improve our overall well-being, and prevent burnout.

Mindfulness Techniques for Stress Reduction

- Mindful Breathing: Deep, intentional breathing can help calm the mind and reduce stress.
- Meditation: Regular meditation practice can reduce stress, anxiety, and depression.
- Mindful Movement: Gentle exercises like yoga and tai chi can help alleviate stress and promote relaxation.
- Mindful Eating: Paying attention to the taste, smell, and texture of food can enhance the eating experience and reduce stress-related eating.
- Mindful Sleep: Establishing a regular sleep routine and practicing mindfulness techniques before bed can improve sleep quality.

By incorporating mindfulness into our daily lives, we can reduce stress, boost our energy levels, and improve our overall quality of life.

Chapter 8
Mindful Communication

Effective communication is essential for building strong relationships and achieving our goals. Mindfulness can significantly enhance our communication skills by helping us to listen actively, express ourselves clearly, and respond thoughtfully.

The Power of Mindful Communication

- Active Listening: By paying full attention to the speaker, we can deepen our understanding and build stronger connections.
- Empathy: Mindfulness can help us develop empathy, the ability to understand and share the feelings of others.
- Non-judgmental Listening: By listening without judgment, we can create a safe and supportive environment for open communication.
- Mindful Speaking: Speaking slowly and clearly, and choosing our words carefully, can help us communicate effectively.
- Assertive Communication: Mindfulness can help us express our needs and wants clearly and assertively.

By practicing mindful communication, we can improve our relationships, resolve conflicts more effectively, and create a more harmonious environment.

Chapter 9
Building Resilience

Resilience is the ability to bounce back from adversity and challenges. It's a crucial skill for navigating life's ups and downs. Mindfulness can significantly enhance our resilience by helping us develop a sense of inner strength, adaptability, and optimism.

Mindfulness and Resilience

- Emotional Regulation: Mindfulness helps us manage our emotions effectively, preventing us from being overwhelmed by stress and negative emotions.
- Positive Reframing: By practicing mindfulness, we can learn to reframe negative experiences in a more positive light.
- Acceptance: Mindfulness encourages us to accept things as they are, rather than resisting or struggling against them.

Mindful Self-Compassion: Treating ourselves with kindness and understanding can boost our resilience.

Practical Tips for Building Resilience

- Mindful Meditation: Regular meditation practice can help cultivate a sense of inner peace and calm.
- Mindful Self-Talk: Replace negative self-talk with positive affirmations.
- Connect with Others: Building strong relationships can provide support and encouragement during challenging times.
- Practice Gratitude: Focusing on the positive aspects of life can boost your mood and outlook.
- Embrace Change: Accept that change is a natural part of life and learn to adapt to new situations.

By incorporating mindfulness into our daily lives, we can develop the resilience needed to overcome obstacles and thrive.

Chapter 10 Mindfulness and Leadership

Mindful leadership is a powerful approach that emphasizes empathy, compassion, and ethical behavior. By cultivating mindfulness, leaders can create positive and productive work environments, inspire their teams, and achieve long-term success.

Key Qualities of
a Mindful Leader

- Self-Awareness: Mindful leaders are aware of their own strengths and weaknesses, as well as their impact on others.
- Emotional Intelligence: They can understand and manage their own emotions, as well as the emotions of their team members.
- Empathy: Mindful leaders are empathetic and compassionate, and they genuinely care about the well-being of their team members.
- Effective Communication: They communicate, concisely, and with empathy.

Ethical Leadership: Mindful leaders adhere to high ethical standards and inspire trust and respect.

Practical Tips for Mindful Leadership

- Mindful Meetings: Conduct meetings with intention and focus.
- Mindful Decision-Making: Make decisions based on reason and compassion.
- Mindful Feedback: Provide constructive feedback in a kind and supportive manner.
- Practice Self-Care: Prioritize self-care to maintain energy and focus.
- Cultivate a Mindful Workplace Culture: Encourage mindfulness practices among team members.

By embodying mindfulness, leaders can create a positive and inspiring work environment that fosters innovation, creativity, and employee satisfaction.

Chapter 11 Achieving Work-Life Balance

Achieving a healthy work-life balance is essential for overall well-being.

Mindfulness can be a powerful tool to help you strike this balance.

Key Strategies for Work-Life Balance

Mindful Time Management:

- Prioritization: Use techniques like the Eisenhower Matrix to prioritize tasks based on urgency and importance.
- Time Blocking: Allocate specific time blocks for work, personal activities, and relaxation.
- Mindful Task Switching: When switching between tasks, take a few moments to transition fully, reducing stress and improving focus.

Mindful Work Habits

- Mindful Multitasking: While multitasking can be tempting, it often leads to decreased productivity and increased stress. Focus on one task at a time.

- Mindful Meetings: Start and end meetings on time, set clear agendas, and actively listen to participants.

Mindful Emailing: Check and respond to emails at specific times, rather than constantly monitoring your inbox.

Mindful Relaxation Techniques

- Meditation: Practice mindfulness meditation to calm the mind and reduce stress.

- Yoga and Pilates: Incorporate these practices into your routine to improve flexibility, strength, and mental clarity.

Spending Time in Nature: Connect with nature through activities like hiking, gardening, or simply spending time outdoors.

Digital Detox

- Screen Time Limits: Set limits on screen time, especially before bed.
- Mindful Social Media Use: Be mindful of the time you spend on social media and the impact it has on your mood.
- Digital Sabbath: Designate specific times to disconnect from technology and focus on other activities.

By incorporating mindfulness into your daily routine, you can achieve a better work-life balance and improve your overall well-being.

Chapter 12
Practical Mindfulness Exercises

Mindfulness doesn't require a retreat or a specific meditation posture. It can be integrated into your daily life through simple exercises. Here are a few to start with:

Mindfulness Meditation:

- Focused Attention Meditation: Direct your attention to a specific object, such as your breath, a mantra, or a physical sensation.
- Open Monitoring Meditation: Allow your thoughts and feelings to arise and pass without judgment.

Loving-Kindness Meditation: Cultivate feelings of love, compassion, and kindness towards yourself and others.

Mindful Movement

- Yoga and Pilates: These practices combine physical postures with breath awareness.
- Tai Chi: A gentle form of exercise that involves slow, flowing movements and deep breathing.

Mindful Walking: Pay attention to the sensation of your feet touching the ground, the rhythm of your breath, and the sights and sounds around you.

Mindful Eating

- Savor Each Bite: Pay attention to the taste, texture, and smell of your food.

- Eat Slowly and Mindfully: Avoid distractions like TV or phones while eating.

Listen to Your Body's Hunger Cues: Eat when you're hungry and stop when you're satisfied.

Mindful Self-Care

- Take Breaks: Schedule regular breaks throughout the day to rest and recharge.

- Practice Gratitude: Focus on the positive aspects of your life.

- Spend Time in Nature: Connect with nature to reduce stress and improve your mood.

By incorporating these practices into your daily routine, you can experience the many benefits of mindfulness. Remember, the key is consistency and patience.

Chapter 13
Advanced Mindfulness Techniques

As you deepen your mindfulness practice, you may explore more advanced techniques to enhance your experience:

Formal Meditation Practices:
- Vipassana Meditation: This technique involves observing sensations in the body without judgment.

- Metta Meditation: Cultivate feelings of loving-kindness towards yourself and others.

Anapanasati Meditation: Focus on the sensation of breath, paying attention to the rise and fall of the breath.

Mindful Inquiry

- Self-Inquiry: Explore your thoughts, feelings, and motivations.

- Journaling: Use journaling to reflect on your experiences and insights.

Mindful Questioning: Ask yourself thoughtful questions to deepen your understanding of yourself and the world.

Mindful Living

- Mindful Work: Incorporate mindfulness into your work practices, such as mindful meetings and mindful email communication.
- Mindful Relationships: Practice active listening, empathy, and non-judgmental communication in your relationships.
- Mindful Parenting: Use mindfulness to connect with your children and respond to their needs with patience and understanding.

Remember, the goal of mindfulness is not to eliminate suffering or negative emotions, but to develop a greater awareness of them. By practicing mindfulness regularly, you can cultivate a greater sense of peace, joy, and well-being.

Chapter 14
Digital Mindfulness

In today's digital age, we are constantly bombarded with information and notifications. This constant stimulation can lead to stress, anxiety, and decreased productivity.

Digital mindfulness is the practice of being present and mindful while using technology.

Strategies for Digital Mindfulness:

Mindful Social Media Use:

- Set Time Limits: Allocate specific time slots for social media.
- Mindful Scrolling: Be intentional about what you consume.

Digital Detox: Take regular breaks from technology.

Mindful Emailing

- Batch Processing: Set specific times to check and respond to emails.

- Mindful Writing: Write clear and concise emails.

Avoid Multitasking: Focus on one task at a time.

Mindful Online Shopping

- Plan Your Purchases: Create a shopping list before browsing online.

Practice Mindful Spending: Avoid impulse purchases.

Mindful Gaming

- Set Time Limits: Limit your gaming time.

- Mindful Gameplay: Focus on the present moment and enjoy the game.

By incorporating these practices into your digital life, you can reduce stress, improve focus, and enhance your overall well-being.

Chapter 15
Mindfulness in Teams

Mindfulness can significantly improve team dynamics, communication, and overall productivity. Here are some ways to incorporate mindfulness into your team:

Mindful Meetings

- Set a Mindful Intention: Begin each meeting with a brief moment of silence or a short meditation to center everyone's attention.
- Active Listening: Encourage active listening by asking clarifying questions and avoiding interruptions.
- Non-Verbal Communication: Pay attention to nonverbal cues like body language and tone of voice.

Mindful Decision-Making: Take time to consider all options and potential consequences before making decisions.

Mindful Communication

- Empathy: Practice empathy by trying to understand others' perspectives.

- Assertive Communication: Express your needs and opinions clearly and respectfully.

Non-Violent Communication: Use "I" statements to express your feelings and needs.

Mindful Conflict Resolution

- Stay Calm: Take a deep breath and count to ten before responding to a conflict.

- Active Listening: Listen to the other person's perspective without interrupting.

Seek Common Ground: Find areas of agreement to build common ground.

Mindful Problem-Solving

- Brainstorming: Encourage creative thinking and open-minded solutions.

- Mindful Decision-Making: Consider all options and potential consequences.

- Learn from Mistakes: Use mistakes as opportunities for growth and learning.

By incorporating mindfulness into your team culture, you can create a more positive, productive, and harmonious work environment.

Chapter 16
Personal Stories
of Mindful Success

Once upon a time, there was a high-powered executive who was constantly juggling work deadlines, client demands, and family responsibilities. The relentless stress had taken a toll on their physical and mental health. They felt overwhelmed, anxious, and unable to relax.

Through mindfulness meditation, this executive learned to slow down, pay attention to their breath, and observe their thoughts without judgment. As they practiced regularly, they noticed a significant shift in their mindset. They became more resilient to stress, more focused on their work, and more patient with their colleagues and family.

The Overwhelmed Parent

A single parent, juggling a demanding job and raising two young children, was feeling constantly overwhelmed. The constant stress and lack of sleep were taking a toll on their physical and mental health. They often felt irritable, impatient, and disconnected from their children.

By incorporating mindfulness practices into their daily routine, these parent learned to manage stress, improve patience, and strengthen their bond with their children. They started their day with a brief meditation session, practiced mindful breathing throughout the day, and engaged in mindful parenting techniques. Through mindfulness, this parent discovered a newfound sense of calm.

The Anxious Student

- A college student experienced high levels of anxiety and difficulty concentrating. Mindfulness techniques helped them to calm their mind, reduce anxiety, and improve academic performance.

These stories illustrate the transformative power of mindfulness. By practicing mindfulness, individuals can experience greater peace, happiness, and success in all areas of their lives.

Chapter 17
Mindfulness in Action
Case Studies

Here are a few case studies demonstrating the positive impact of mindfulness in various settings:

1. Mindfulness in the Workplace

- Increased Productivity: A tech company implemented mindfulness programs for its employees, leading to increased productivity, reduced stress, and improved job satisfaction.

Enhanced Creativity: An advertising agency introduced mindfulness meditation into its daily routine, leading to more creative and innovative campaigns.

2. Mindfulness in Healthcare

- Reduced Patient Anxiety: Hospitals and clinics have used mindfulness techniques to reduce patient anxiety and improve the overall patient experience.

Improved Healthcare Worker Well-being: Mindfulness programs for healthcare professionals have been shown to reduce burnout, improve job satisfaction, and enhance patient care.

3. Mindfulness in Education

- Improved Student Performance: Schools and universities have incorporated mindfulness into their curriculum, leading to improved student focus, concentration, and academic performance.

Enhanced Teacher Well-being: Mindfulness practices have helped teachers manage stress, improve classroom management, and create a more positive learning environment.

4. Mindfulness in the Criminal Justice System

- Reduced Recidivism: Mindfulness-based programs in prisons have been shown to reduce recidivism rates by teaching inmates stress management, emotional regulation, and conflict resolution skills.

These case studies highlight the versatility of mindfulness and its potential to positively impact individuals and organizations across various sectors.

Chapter 18
Addressing Skepticism
and
Misunderstandings

While mindfulness has gained significant popularity, it's not without its critics. Here are some common misconceptions and how to address them:

Misconception 1
Mindfulness is a Religious Practice

Reality: Mindfulness is a secular practice that can be adapted to fit various belief systems. It's about paying attention to the present moment without judgment.

Misconception 2
Mindfulness is Only for Stress Reduction

Reality: While mindfulness is effective for stress reduction, its benefits extend far beyond that. It can enhance focus, creativity, emotional intelligence, and overall well-being.

Misconception 3
Mindfulness Takes
Too Much Time

Reality: Even short periods of mindfulness practice can have significant benefits. You can practice mindfulness for a few minutes each day, or even incorporate it into your daily activities.

Misconception 4
Mindfulness
is Not Practical in the
Real World

Reality: Mindfulness can be applied to various aspects of your life, including work, relationships, and parenting. By practicing mindfulness, you can develop greater self-awareness, empathy, and resilience.

Misconception 5
Mindfulness is Only for Experienced Meditators

- **Reality:** Mindfulness is accessible to everyone, regardless of experience or background. There are many simple techniques that you can start practicing today.

By addressing these common misconceptions, we can encourage more people to explore the benefits of mindfulness and incorporate it into their daily lives.

Chapter 19
Cultivating
a Lifelong Mindful Practice

Cultivating a lifelong mindfulness practice requires dedication and consistency. Here are some tips to help you stay on track:

- **Set Realistic Goals:** Start with small, achievable goals and gradually increase your practice time.

Find a Supportive Community: Join a mindfulness group or find a meditation partner to share your experiences and stay motivated.

- **Make Mindfulness a Daily Habit:** Incorporate mindfulness into your daily routine, such as practicing mindfulness during your morning routine or before bed.

- **Be Patient and Kind to Yourself:** Remember that progress takes time. Don't get discouraged if you have setbacks.

- **Seek Guidance:** Consider working with a mindfulness teacher or therapist to deepen your practice.

- **Integrate Mindfulness into Your Life:** Apply mindfulness to all areas of your life, including work, relationships, and leisure activities.

By following these tips, you can develop a sustainable mindfulness practice that will benefit you for years to come.

Chapter 20
The Future of Mindfulness and Success

The future of mindfulness is bright. As more research emerges and mindfulness becomes more widely accepted, we can expect to see its integration into various aspects of our lives, including education, healthcare, and business.

Here are some potential trends and innovations in the field of mindfulness

- **Mindfulness Technology:** The development of mindfulness apps and wearable devices that can track and improve mindfulness practices.
- **Mindful Education:** The integration of mindfulness into school curricula to improve student focus, creativity, and emotional intelligence.
- **Mindful Workplace Culture:** The creation of mindfulness-based workplaces that promote employee well-being and productivity.
- **Mindful Healthcare:** The use of mindfulness techniques to reduce stress, anxiety, and pain in healthcare settings.

By embracing mindfulness, we can create a more compassionate, sustainable, and fulfilling future for ourselves for the planet.

Conclusion
A Mindful Journey

As we conclude this journey into the world of mindfulness, it's clear that this ancient practice offers a powerful tool for navigating the complexities of modern life. By cultivating mindfulness, we can unlock our full potential, enhance our relationships, and experience greater peace and joy. Remember, the key to a successful mindfulness practice is consistency and patience. Start small and gradually increase your practice time. Don't be afraid to experiment with different techniques and find what works best for you.

By integrating mindfulness into your daily life, you can create a more mindful, compassionate, and fulfilling existence. Embrace the journey, and may your path be filled with peace and prosperity.

Mentions

Books:

- Full Catastrophe Living by Jon Kabat-Zinn
- Mindfulness in Plain English by Henepola Gunaratana
- Wherever You Go, There You Are by Jon Kabat-Zinn
- Search Inside Yourself by Chade-Meng Tan
- The Power of Now by Eckhart Tolle
- Research Papers and Articles:

Mindfulness-Based Stress Reduction (MBSR): A well-researched program developed by Jon Kabat-Zinn. Numerous studies have demonstrated its effectiveness in reducing stress, anxiety, and depression.

- Neuroimaging Studies: Research using fMRI and other neuroimaging techniques has shown that mindfulness practices can alter brain structure and function, particularly in areas related to attention, emotion regulation, and self-awareness.

Meta-Analyses of Mindfulness Research: Several meta-analyses have synthesized the results of numerous studies, providing strong evidence for the benefits of mindfulness in various areas of life.

Additional Resources

- American Psychological Association (APA): The APA has published numerous articles and reports on the benefits of mindfulness.

- National Center for Complementary and Integrative Health (NCCIH): The NCCIH provides information on the science of mindfulness and its potential health benefits.

Mindfulness-Based Stress Reduction Clinics: These clinics offer mindfulness-based programs and can provide additional resources and guidance.

Please note that it's important to consult with a healthcare professional before starting any new mindfulness practice, especially if you have underlying health conditions.

References

- Kabat-Zinn, J. (1994). Full catastrophe living: How to cope with stress, pain, and illness using mindfulness meditation. Dell Publishing.
- Kabat-Zinn, J. (2005). Wherever You Go, There You Are: Mindfulness Meditation in Everyday Life. Hyperion.
- Siegel, D. J. (2010). Mindsight: The New Science of Personal Transformation. Bantam Books.
- Goleman, D. (2006). Emotional Intelligence: Why It Can Matter More Than IQ. Bantam Books.
- Brown, B. (2013). Daring Greatly: How to Courageously Live a Wholehearted Life. Hazelden Publishing.

- Davidson, R. J., & Begley, S. (2012). The mindful brain: Reflection and attunement in the age of the stressed brain. Avery.
- Hanson, R. (2013). Buddha's Brain: The Practical Neuroscience of Happiness, Love, and Wisdom. New Harbinger Publications.
- Germer, C. K., Siegel, R. D., & Davidson, R. J. (2013). Mindfulness and Psychotherapy. Guilford Press.
- Shapiro, S. L., Carlson, L. E., Astin, J. A., & Freedman, B. (2006). Mindfulness-based stress reduction for health care professionals: Results from a randomized controlled trial. Journal of Consulting and Clinical Psychology, 74(2), 164-176.
- Chiesa, A., Serretti, A., & Merla, A. (2011). Mindfulness-based interventions for stress reduction and well-being: A systematic review and meta-analysis. Psychotherapy and Psychosomatics, 80(2), 104-114.

- Keng, S. L., Smoski, M. J., & Leary, M. R. (2011). Mindfulness meditation and anxiety: A meta-analysis of randomized controlled trials. Depression and Anxiety, 28(8), 623-631.
- Hofmann, S. G., Sawyer, A. T., Witt, A. A., & Hayes, S. C. (2010). The mindful way through depression: Freeing the mind from chronic sadness. Guilford Press.
- Kabat-Zinn, J. (2012). Full Catastrophe Living: How to Cope with Stress, Pain, and Illness Using Mindfulness Meditation. Penguin Books.
- Williams, J. M. G., & Penman, D. (2011). Mindfulness: An eight-week plan for finding peace in a frantic world. Random House.
- Gottfredson, N. (2015). Mindfulness in Seven Minutes: A Practical Guide to Finding Peace in Your Day. HarperOne.
- Hayes, S. C., Strosahl, K. D., & Wilson, K. G. (1999). Acceptance and Commitment Therapy: An Experiential Approach to Behavior Change. Guilford Press.
-
- Neff, K. D. (2011). Self-Compassion: The Proven Power of Being Kind to Yourself. William Morrow.
- Langer, E. J. (2009). Mindfulness. Da Capo Press.
- Chödrön, P. (2001). The Places That Scare You: A Guide to Fearlessness in Difficult Times. Shambhala Publications.
- Tolle, E. (2004). The Power of Now: A Guide to Spiritual Enlightenment. New World Library.

www.ingramcontent.com/pod-product-compliance
Lightning Source LLC
Chambersburg PA
CBHW071558270726
48657CB00026B/783